# DASH DIET COOKBOOK FOR BEGINNERS 2024

Discover the Keys to Reducing Blood Pressure and Embracing Vibrant Health with Fast, Delicious Meals

**By**

## Hector Wiggins

# Table of Contents

# CHAPTER ONE

## Introduction

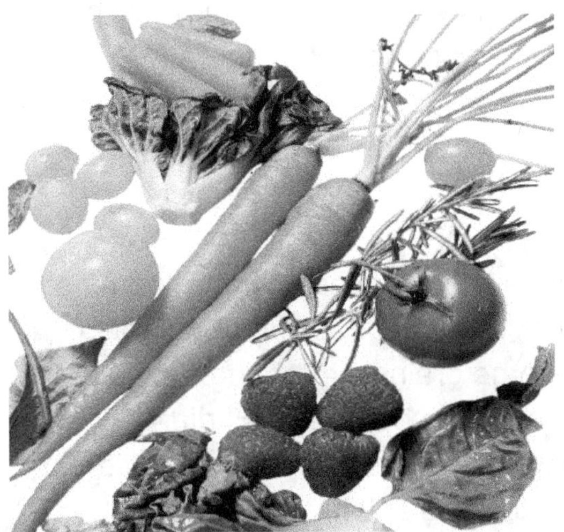

In a world where fad diets come and go like fleeting trends, the DASH (Dietary Approaches to Stop Hypertension) diet stands out as a beacon of balanced nutrition and sustainable lifestyle change.

More than just a passing craze, the DASH diet
has garnered praise from health experts and
individuals alike for its effectiveness in lowering
blood pressure, promoting heart health, and
fostering overall well-being. And now, with the
"Dash Diet Cookbook for Beginners,"
embarking on this journey towards better
health has never been more accessible or
delicious.

Picture this: a kitchen filled with the aroma of
freshly chopped herbs, sizzling vegetables,
and wholesome grains simmering on the stove.
This is the essence of the DASH diet—a
culinary adventure that celebrates the vibrant
flavors of whole foods while prioritizing
nutrient-rich ingredients that nourish the body
from within. But beyond its culinary appeal, the
DASH diet represents a paradigm shift in the
way we approach food—a departure from
restrictive eating patterns towards a more
holistic and sustainable approach to nutrition.

So, what exactly is the DASH diet, and why has it captured the attention of health-conscious individuals around the globe? At its core, the DASH diet emphasizes a balanced approach to eating, focusing on whole foods such as fruits, vegetables, lean proteins, and whole grains while minimizing the consumption of sodium, saturated fats, and processed foods. This approach not only helps to lower blood pressure but also contributes to weight management, reduces the risk of chronic diseases, and promotes overall vitality.

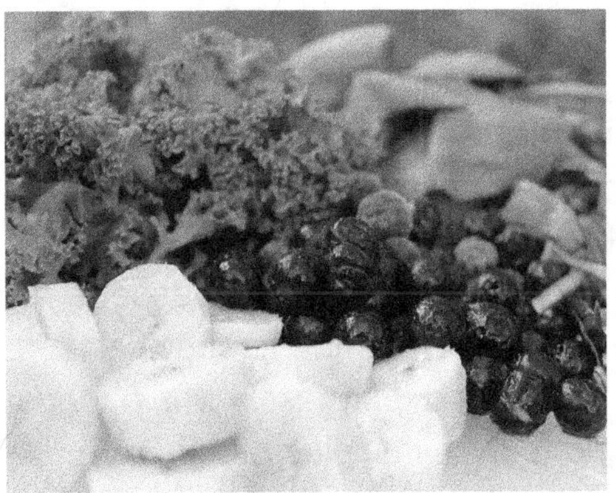

But here's the best part: the "Dash Diet Cookbook for Beginners" takes the guesswork out of adopting this lifestyle, offering a comprehensive guide filled with delicious recipes, practical tips, and expert advice to help you navigate your journey towards better health with confidence and ease. Whether you're a seasoned home cook or a novice in the kitchen, this cookbook provides everything you need to get started on the DASH diet, from pantry staples and kitchen essentials to meal planning strategies and cooking techniques.

Imagine flipping through the pages of this cookbook and discovering a treasure trove of culinary inspiration at your fingertips. From hearty breakfasts to satisfying lunches, wholesome dinners, and decadent desserts, each recipe is carefully crafted to showcase the diverse flavors and textures of whole foods while adhering to the principles of the DASH diet.

Whether you're craving a comforting bowl of oatmeal topped with fresh berries, a colorful salad bursting with seasonal vegetables, or a flavorful stir-fry packed with lean protein and vibrant spices, there's something for everyone to enjoy.

But the "Dash Diet Cookbook for Beginners" is more than just a collection of recipes—it's a roadmap to a healthier, happier you. With its practical approach to meal planning, shopping guides, and meal prep strategies, this cookbook empowers you to take control of your health and well-being one delicious bite at a time. Whether you're looking to lower your blood pressure, shed unwanted pounds, or simply adopt a more balanced approach to eating, the DASH diet offers a pathway to success that is both sustainable and satisfying.

So, are you ready to embark on this culinary journey towards better health? With the "Dash Diet Cookbook for Beginners" as your guide, the possibilities are endless. Get ready to savor the flavors of wholesome, nourishing foods, revitalize your health, and transform your life—one delicious recipe at a time.

## What is the DASH Diet?

The DASH (Dietary Approaches to Stop
Hypertension) diet is a dietary pattern
recognized for its effectiveness in reducing
blood pressure and promoting overall heart
health. Developed by the National Heart, Lung,
and Blood Institute (NHLBI), the DASH diet
was originally designed to prevent and manage
hypertension, but it has since gained popularity
for its broader health benefits.

At its core, the DASH diet emphasizes
consuming a variety of nutrient-rich foods while
limiting the intake of sodium, saturated fats,
and added sugars. It is based on research
showing that certain dietary components can
significantly impact blood pressure levels and
cardiovascular health.

**The primary components of the DASH diet include:**

**Fruits and vegetables**: Packed with vitamins, minerals, and antioxidants, fruits and vegetables are recommended as a major part of the DASH diet. These foods support general hydration and fullness in addition to offering vital nutrients.

**Whole grains:** Whole grains are a key source of fiber, which can help regulate blood sugar levels and promote digestive health. The DASH diet recommends incorporating whole grains such as brown rice, quinoa, oats, and whole wheat into meals and snacks.

**Lean proteins:** Lean protein sources, such as poultry, fish, beans, and legumes, are prioritized in the DASH diet. These foods provide essential amino acids while being lower in saturated fat compared to red meat and processed meats.

**Low-fat dairy**: Dairy products are included in the DASH diet, but emphasis is placed on choosing low-fat or fat-free options to reduce saturated fat intake. Calcium-rich foods like milk, yogurt, and cheese can support bone health and provide essential nutrients.

**Limited sodium:** Excessive sodium intake is known to elevate blood pressure, so the DASH diet recommends limiting salt intake to no more than 2,300 milligrams per day. This can be achieved by choosing fresh or minimally processed foods, using herbs and spices for flavoring, and avoiding high-sodium condiments and processed snacks.

**Limited saturated fats and added sugars:** Foods high in saturated fats and added sugars, such as fried foods, sweets, and sugary beverages, should be consumed in moderation on the DASH diet. Instead, emphasis is placed on healthier fats like those found in nuts, seeds, and olive oil, as well as natural sources of sweetness like fruits.

Overall, the DASH diet promotes a balanced and varied approach to eating that emphasizes nutrient-dense foods and minimizes the consumption of unhealthy ingredients. By following the principles of the DASH diet, individuals can not only lower their blood pressure but also reduce their risk of developing chronic diseases such as heart disease, stroke, and diabetes.

# Benefits of the DASH Diet

The DASH (Dietary Approaches to Stop Hypertension) diet is well-known for its health benefits.
These health benefits includes:

**Lowers Blood Pressure**: The primary goal of the DASH diet is to reduce blood pressure. It emphasizes foods rich in potassium, calcium, magnesium, and fiber, which have been shown to help lower blood pressure.

**Reduces Risk of Heart Disease**: By promoting heart-healthy foods like fruits, vegetables, whole grains, and lean proteins, the DASH diet can lower the risk of heart disease and improve overall cardiovascular health.

**Aids Weight Loss:** The DASH diet encourages portion control and emphasizes nutrient-dense foods, making it effective for weight management and promoting a healthy body weight.

**Improves Cholesterol Levels**: The diet's emphasis on whole grains, fruits, vegetables, and lean proteins can help improve cholesterol levels, reducing the risk of heart disease and stroke.

**Promotes Healthy Digestion:** The high fiber content of the DASH diet, derived from fruits, vegetables, and whole grains, supports healthy digestion and may reduce the risk of digestive issues such as constipation and diverticulosis.

**Manages Diabetes**: The DASH diet's focus on whole foods, low in saturated fats and added sugars, can help manage blood sugar levels and improve insulin sensitivity, making it beneficial for individuals with diabetes.

**Supports Bone Health**: The inclusion of calcium-rich foods like dairy products and fortified foods in the DASH diet helps support bone health and may reduce the risk of osteoporosis.

**Reduces Cancer Risk**: The abundance of fruits, vegetables, and whole grains in the DASH diet provides a variety of antioxidants and phytochemicals that may help reduce the risk of certain cancers, such as colorectal cancer.

**Improves Overall Nutritional Intake:** By promoting a balanced diet rich in vitamins, minerals, and other essential nutrients, the DASH diet supports overall health and well-being, reducing the risk of nutrient deficiencies.

**Easy to Follow and Sustainable**: The DASH diet emphasizes whole, nutrient-dense foods that are readily available and easy to incorporate into daily meals, making it a practical and sustainable approach to healthy eating for the long term.

# How the DASH Diet Works

The DASH (Dietary Approaches to Stop Hypertension) diet is designed to lower blood pressure and improve overall health by promoting a balanced and nutritious eating pattern. Here's a comprehensive explanation of how the DASH diet works:

**Emphasis on Nutrient-Rich Foods**: The DASH diet emphasizes foods that are rich in nutrients such as potassium, calcium, magnesium, and fiber. These nutrients have been shown to have beneficial effects on blood pressure regulation and overall cardiovascular health.

**Reduction of Sodium Intake:** One of the key principles of the DASH diet is to reduce sodium intake, as high sodium consumption is associated with elevated blood pressure. The diet recommends limiting sodium to no more than 2,300 milligrams per day, with an ideal target of 1,500 milligrams per day for even greater blood pressure reduction.

**Emphasis on Fruits and Vegetables**: Packed with dietary fiber, vitamins, minerals, and antioxidants, a variety of fruits and vegetables are recommended as part of the DASH diet. These meals promote general heart health by lowering blood pressure and reducing inflammation.

**Inclusion of Whole Grains**: Whole grains, such as brown rice, quinoa, oats, and whole wheat, are a staple of the DASH diet. They provide essential nutrients and fiber, which help regulate blood sugar levels, promote satiety, and contribute to overall cardiovascular health.

**Lean Protein Sources:** The DASH diet includes lean protein sources such as poultry, fish, beans, nuts, and legumes, while limiting red meat consumption. These protein sources are lower in saturated fat and cholesterol, making them heart-healthy choices.

**Moderate Dairy Intake**: The DASH diet includes low-fat or fat-free dairy products such as milk, yogurt, and cheese. These foods are rich in calcium and vitamin D, which are essential for bone health and may also help lower blood pressure.

**Healthy Fats:** While the DASH diet emphasizes reducing saturated fats and trans fats, it encourages the consumption of healthy fats found in foods like avocados, nuts, seeds, and olive oil. These fats have been shown to have beneficial effects on heart health and may help lower blood pressure.

**Portion Control and Balanced Meals**: The DASH diet promotes portion control and balanced meals, with an emphasis on eating smaller, more frequent meals throughout the day. By controlling portion sizes and distributing nutrients evenly across meals, the diet helps maintain stable blood sugar levels and promotes overall well-being.

**Regular Physical Activity**: While not specifically a dietary component, regular physical activity is an important part of the DASH diet plan. Exercise helps lower blood pressure, improve cardiovascular health, and enhance overall fitness, complementing the dietary strategies of the DASH diet.

**Lifestyle Modification**: In addition to dietary changes, the DASH diet encourages lifestyle modifications such as managing stress, quitting smoking, limiting alcohol consumption, and getting an adequate amount of sleep. These lifestyle factors play a crucial role in maintaining optimal blood pressure and overall health.

# Getting Started: Tips for Success

Getting started with the DASH diet can be made easier with the help of a DASH diet cookbook. Here's a comprehensive discussion on tips for success when using a DASH diet cookbook:

**Selecting the Right Cookbook**: Choose a DASH diet cookbook that suits your preferences and dietary needs. Look for cookbooks with a variety of recipes, clear instructions, and nutritional information. Consider whether you prefer traditional printed cookbooks or digital versions, as well as any specific dietary considerations such as vegetarian, gluten-free, or dairy-free options.

**Understanding the DASH Diet Principles:** Before diving into the recipes, take some time to familiarize yourself with the principles of the DASH diet. Understand the importance of consuming nutrient-rich foods, limiting sodium intake, and incorporating a variety of fruits, vegetables, whole grains, lean proteins, and healthy fats into your meals.

**Meal Planning and Preparation**: Plan your meals in advance using the recipes provided in the cookbook. Create a weekly meal plan that includes a balance of different food groups and flavors. Take into account your schedule, preferences, and any dietary restrictions or allergies. Make a shopping list based on the ingredients needed for the recipes, and ensure you have the necessary kitchen equipment and pantry staples on hand.

**Start Simple:** Begin with simple and familiar recipes to ease into the DASH diet lifestyle. Look for recipes that require minimal ingredients and preparation time, such as salads, soups, stir-fries, and one-pot meals. Gradually experiment with more complex recipes as you become more comfortable with the cooking techniques and flavor combinations.

**Focus on Flavor**: The DASH diet doesn't mean sacrificing flavor. Experiment with herbs, spices, citrus, and other seasonings to enhance the taste of your meals without relying on excessive salt or sodium-laden condiments. Many DASH diet cookbooks offer flavor-packed recipes that showcase the natural flavors of wholesome ingredients.

**Portion Control**: Pay attention to portion sizes when preparing and serving your meals. Use measuring cups, spoons, and kitchen scales to accurately portion out ingredients and avoid overeating. The DASH diet emphasizes eating smaller, more frequent meals throughout the day to help regulate blood sugar levels and promote satiety.

**Flexibility and Variety**: Try new recipes and ingredients on a regular basis to keep your meals interesting and varied. Never hesitate to alter recipes to accommodate your dietary restrictions or personal tastes. A lot of DASH diet cookbooks provide suggestions for customizing meals to fit a variety of tastes and dietary constraints.

**Stay Consistent and Patient**: Consistency is key to success with the DASH diet. Stick to your meal plan, and don't get discouraged by setbacks or occasional indulgences. It may take time to adjust to the new eating pattern and see noticeable improvements in your health, so be patient and stay committed to your goals.

**Seek Support and Resources**: Consider joining online forums, social media groups, or local DASH diet support groups to connect with others following the same dietary guidelines. Share recipe ideas, meal planning tips, and success stories to stay motivated and inspired on your DASH diet journey. Utilize additional resources such as websites, apps, and cooking classes to expand your knowledge and culinary skills.

**Monitor Progress and Adjust as Needed**: Keep track of your progress by monitoring your blood pressure, weight, energy levels, and overall well-being. If necessary, consult with a healthcare professional or registered dietitian for personalized guidance and adjustments to your DASH diet plan. Stay open-minded and willing to adapt your approach based on your individual needs and feedback from your body.

# CHAPTER TWO

## Understanding the DASH Diet Principles

The DASH (Dietary Approaches to Stop Hypertension) diet is based on several key principles aimed at promoting overall health and lowering blood pressure. Here's a comprehensive explanation of the DASH diet principles:

**Emphasis on Nutrient-Rich Foods:** The DASH diet encourages the consumption of foods that are rich in essential nutrients such as potassium, calcium, magnesium, and fiber. These nutrients play crucial roles in regulating blood pressure, supporting cardiovascular health, and promoting overall well-being.

**High Intake of Fruits and Vegetables:** Fruits and vegetables are central to the DASH diet and should form a significant portion of daily food intake. These foods are rich in vitamins, minerals, antioxidants, and dietary fiber, which help lower blood pressure, reduce inflammation, and support heart health.

**Whole Grains as Staples**: Whole grains such as brown rice, quinoa, oats, barley, and whole wheat are encouraged on the DASH diet. These grains provide essential nutrients and fiber while also helping to regulate blood sugar levels and promote satiety.

**Lean Protein Sources:** The DASH diet promotes lean protein sources such as poultry, fish, beans, nuts, and legumes. These protein sources are lower in saturated fat and cholesterol compared to red meat, making them heart-healthy choices. They also provide important nutrients like iron and zinc.

**Limited Sodium Intake**: Excessive sodium intake is linked to high blood pressure, so the DASH diet recommends limiting sodium consumption. The diet suggests consuming no more than 2,300 milligrams of sodium per day, with an ideal target of 1,500 milligrams per day for even greater blood pressure reduction.

**Moderate Dairy Products**: The DASH diet includes low-fat or fat-free dairy products such as milk, yogurt, and cheese. These foods are excellent sources of calcium and vitamin D, which are essential for bone health. However, portion sizes should be moderate to avoid excessive saturated fat intake.

**Healthy Fats in Moderation**: While the DASH diet emphasizes reducing saturated and trans fats, it encourages the consumption of healthy fats found in foods like avocados, nuts, seeds, and olive oil. These fats have been shown to have beneficial effects on heart health when consumed in moderation.

**Portion Control and Balanced Meals**: Portion control is essential on the DASH diet to prevent overeating and maintain a healthy weight. Meals should be balanced and include a variety of nutrient-rich foods from different food groups, such as fruits, vegetables, whole grains, lean proteins, and healthy fats.

**Regular Physical Activity**: In addition to dietary changes, the DASH diet recommends regular physical activity as part of a healthy lifestyle. Exercise helps lower blood pressure, improve cardiovascular health, and contribute to overall well-being.

**Lifestyle Modification**: Beyond diet and exercise, the DASH diet emphasizes lifestyle modifications such as managing stress, quitting smoking, limiting alcohol consumption, and getting adequate sleep. These lifestyle factors play a crucial role in maintaining optimal blood pressure and overall health.

# Key Components of the DASH Diet

The DASH (Dietary Approaches to Stop Hypertension) diet consists of key components that form the foundation of its approach to promoting overall health and lowering blood pressure.

These components includes:

**Fruits and Vegetables**: Fruits and vegetables are central to the DASH diet. They are rich in vitamins, minerals, antioxidants, and dietary fiber, which help lower blood pressure, reduce inflammation, and support heart health. Aim for at least 4-5 servings of fruits and 4-5 servings of vegetables per day.

**Whole Grains:** Whole grains help control blood sugar levels, increase satiety, and supply fiber and vital nutrients. Brown rice, quinoa, oats, barley, and whole wheat bread are a few types of whole grains. Include six to eight servings of whole grains in your daily diet.

**Low-Fat or Fat-Free Dairy Products**: Low-fat or fat-free dairy products such as milk, yogurt, and cheese are important sources of calcium and vitamin D, which are essential for bone health. Choose dairy products that are low in saturated fat and limit portions to 2-3 servings per day.

**Limited Sodium Intake**: The DASH diet advises decreasing sodium consumption since too much sodium is associated with elevated blood pressure. Limit your daily salt intake to a maximum of 2,300 mg, ideally staying below 1,500 mg to further lower blood pressure.

**Healthy Fats:** While the DASH diet emphasizes reducing saturated and trans fats, it encourages the consumption of healthy fats found in foods like avocados, nuts, seeds, and olive oil. These fats have been shown to have beneficial effects on heart health when consumed in moderation.

**Portion Control**: Portion control is essential on the DASH diet to prevent overeating and maintain a healthy weight. Be mindful of serving sizes and avoid oversized portions, especially of calorie-dense foods.

**Balanced Meals**: Meals should be balanced and include a variety of nutrient-rich foods from different food groups. Aim to include fruits, vegetables, whole grains, lean proteins, and healthy fats in each meal to ensure you're getting a wide range of essential nutrients.

**Frequent Physical exercise**: As part of a healthy lifestyle, the DASH diet advocates regular physical exercise in addition to food modifications. Exercise promotes cardiovascular health, lowers blood pressure, and enhances general wellbeing.

# Recommended Servings and Portions

The DASH (Dietary Approaches to Stop Hypertension) diet is a dietary pattern that emphasizes consuming nutrient-rich foods to help lower blood pressure and improve overall health. Here's a comprehensive breakdown of the recommended servings and portions for the DASH diet:

**Vegetables:** Aim for 4-5 servings per day. Vegetables are rich in vitamins, minerals, fiber, and antioxidants, making them essential for overall health. Include a variety of colorful vegetables such as leafy greens, carrots, bell peppers, broccoli, and tomatoes to ensure a diverse nutrient intake.

**Fruits**: Aim for three to four servings daily. In addition, fruits are a great source of fiber, antioxidants, vitamins, and minerals. To reach your recommended intake, include a selection of fruits in your daily meals and snacks, such as berries, oranges, apples, bananas, and melons.

**Grains:** Focus on whole grains and aim for 6–8 servings daily. Fiber, B vitamins, and minerals like iron and magnesium are all found in whole grains. Brown rice, quinoa, oats, barley, and whole wheat bread or pasta are a few types of whole grains. Refined grains, which have less fiber and nutrients, should be avoided. Examples of these are white bread and rice.

**Lean protein sources**: Aim for 2 or fewer servings per day. Choose lean protein sources such as poultry (without skin), fish, beans, lentils, tofu, and nuts. These foods provide protein, essential amino acids, vitamins, and minerals while being lower in saturated fat compared to red and processed meats.

**Low-fat or fat-free dairy products**: Aim for 2-3 servings per day. Dairy products are excellent sources of calcium, vitamin D, and protein. Opt for low-fat or fat-free options such as skim milk, yogurt, and cheese to reduce saturated fat intake. If you're lactose intolerant or prefer non-dairy alternatives, fortified soy milk or almond milk can be suitable substitutes.

**Fats and oils**: Limit intake. While fats are essential for overall health, it's important to consume them in moderation, especially sources high in saturated and trans fats. Choose healthier fats such as olive oil, avocado, nuts, and seeds, and limit butter, margarine, and high-fat condiments.

**Sweets and added sugars**: Limit intake. Foods and beverages high in added sugars contribute excess calories and offer little nutritional value. Limit desserts, sugary snacks, sodas, and sweetened beverages, and opt for natural sources of sweetness such as fruits or small amounts of honey or maple syrup when needed.

In summary, the DASH diet emphasizes consuming a variety of nutrient-rich foods in appropriate portions to support overall health and manage blood pressure. By following these recommendations, individuals can create balanced and satisfying meals while promoting heart health and overall well-being. Additionally, incorporating regular physical activity and maintaining a healthy weight are important compliments to the DASH diet for optimal health outcomes.

# Understanding Sodium Intake

Understanding sodium intake is crucial when following the DASH (Dietary Approaches to Stop Hypertension) diet, as excessive sodium consumption is linked to high blood pressure and cardiovascular disease. Here's a comprehensive explanation of sodium intake in the context of the DASH diet:

**Recommended Sodium Levels:** The DASH diet recommends limiting sodium intake to no more than 2,300 milligrams (mg) per day, with an ideal target of 1,500 mg per day for most adults, especially those with hypertension or at risk of developing it. This lower target can significantly reduce blood pressure and lower the risk of heart disease.

**Sources of Sodium**: Sodium is naturally present in many foods, but it's also added during processing, cooking, and at the table.

The main sources of dietary sodium include processed and packaged foods, canned soups and vegetables, deli meats, cheese, bread, condiments, and fast food. Monitoring sodium content on food labels and choosing lower-sodium options can help reduce intake.

**Effects of Excessive Sodium Intake**: High sodium intake can lead to fluid retention, increased blood volume, and elevated blood pressure, putting strain on the heart and blood vessels. Over time, this can contribute to the development of hypertension, stroke, heart disease, kidney damage, and other health complications. Reducing sodium intake is essential for managing and preventing these conditions.

**Tips for Reducing Sodium Intake:**

**Select fresh, complete foods**: Increase your intake of fruits, vegetables, whole grains, lean meats, and low-fat dairy products. These foods are high in nutrients and naturally low in salt.

**Read food labels:** Check the sodium content on packaged foods and choose products labeled "low-sodium," "reduced sodium," or "no added salt" whenever possible.

**Use herbs and spices:** Enhance the flavor of your meals with herbs, spices, citrus juices, vinegar, and other flavorings instead of salt.

**Cook at home:** Prepare meals from scratch using fresh ingredients to have more control over the sodium content of your food.

**Limit processed and restaurant foods:** Minimize consumption of processed snacks, fast food, restaurant meals, and takeout, as these tend to be high in sodium.

Use sauces, condiments, and salad dressings sparingly because they can be substantial sources of unrecognized salt.

**Gradual Reduction**: If you're accustomed to a high-sodium diet, aim to gradually reduce your intake over time to allow your taste buds to adjust to lower sodium levels. This approach can make the transition easier and more sustainable.

In summary, understanding sodium intake is essential for effectively following the DASH diet and promoting heart health. By monitoring sodium levels, choosing lower-sodium options, and incorporating fresh, whole foods into your diet, you can lower blood pressure, reduce the risk of cardiovascular disease, and improve overall well-being.

# CHAPTER THREE

## Stocking Your Kitchen for Success

Stocking your kitchen for success on the DASH diet is essential for maintaining a healthy and balanced eating plan. The DASH diet, which stands for Dietary Approaches to Stop Hypertension, is a popular eating plan that focuses on reducing sodium intake and increasing consumption of fruits, vegetables, whole grains, and lean proteins. By stocking your kitchen with the right ingredients, you can easily prepare nutritious meals that align with the principles of the DASH diet.

**Here are some tips for stocking your kitchen for success on the DASH diet:**

1. **Fruits and vegetables**: Make sure to have a variety of fresh, frozen, and canned fruits and vegetables on hand. Option for colorful options

like berries, leafy greens, bell peppers, and sweet potatoes. These foods are rich in vitamins, minerals, and antioxidants that support overall health and help lower blood pressure.

2. **Whole grains**: Choose whole grain options like brown rice, quinoa, whole wheat pasta, and oats. These foods are high in fiber, which can help lower cholesterol levels and improve heart health. Avoid refined grains like white bread and white rice, which are lower in nutrients.

3. **Lean proteins**: Stock up on lean protein sources like skinless poultry, fish, tofu, beans, and lentils. These foods are lower in saturated fat and cholesterol compared to red meat and processed meats. Aim to include protein in every meal to help you feel full and satisfied.

4. **Dairy**: Option for low-fat or fat-free dairy products like milk, yogurt, and cheese. These foods are good sources of calcium and protein, which are important for bone health and muscle function. Choose plain or unsweetened options to avoid added sugars.

5. **Nuts and seeds**: Keep a variety of nuts and seeds on hand for snacking or adding to meals. Nuts like almonds, walnuts, and pistachios are rich in heart-healthy fats, protein, and fiber. Seeds like chia, flax, and pumpkin seeds are also good sources of nutrients.

6. **Herbs and spices:** Enhance the flavor of your meals with herbs and spices instead of salt. Stock your pantry with options like garlic, basil, oregano, cinnamon, and turmeric. These ingredients can add depth and complexity to your dishes without adding extra sodium.

7. **Healthy fats:** Include sources of healthy fats in your kitchen like olive oil, avocado, and fatty fish. These foods contain omega-3 fatty acids, which have been shown to reduce inflammation and improve heart health. Use olive oil for cooking and salad dressings, and add avocado to smoothies, salads, or sandwiches.

By stocking your kitchen with these nutritious ingredients, you can easily prepare meals that align with the principles of the DASH diet. Remember to plan ahead, make a grocery list, and prioritize whole, minimally processed foods to support your health and well-being. With a well-stocked kitchen, you'll be well-equipped to follow the DASH diet and achieve your health goals.

# Essential Ingredients for the DASH Diet

A dietary regimen called the DASH (Dietary Approaches to Stop Hypertension) diet is intended to help decrease blood pressure and enhance heart health in general. It places a strong emphasis on eating a range of foods high in nutrients and low in saturated fats and salt. Among the DASH diet's most crucial components are the following:

**Fruits and veggies**: Packed with vitamins, minerals, and antioxidants, fruits and vegetables can help lower blood pressure and reduce inflammation. They can aid in weight management because they are high in fiber and low in calories.

**Whole grains**: Whole grains, such as brown rice, quinoa, and whole wheat bread, are high in fiber and nutrients that can help lower cholesterol levels and improve heart health.

**Lean proteins:** Lean proteins, such as chicken, fish, and beans, are important for muscle growth and repair. They are also lower in saturated fats, which can help reduce the risk of heart disease.

**Dairy products**: Low-fat or fat-free dairy products, such as milk, yogurt, and cheese, are good sources of calcium and vitamin D, which are important for bone health. They also provide protein and other essential nutrients.

**Nuts and seeds**: Nuts and seeds are high in healthy fats, protein, and fiber, which can help lower cholesterol levels and reduce the risk of heart disease.

**Healthy fats:** Nuts, avocados, and olive oil are good sources of healthy fats that are crucial for lowering inflammation in the body and supporting brain function. They can also strengthen heart health and decrease cholesterol.

# Kitchen Tools and Equipment

To successfully follow the DASH (Dietary Approaches to Stop Hypertension) diet, having the right kitchen tools and equipment can make meal preparation easier and more enjoyable. Here are some necessary kitchen tools and equipment for the DASH diet:

**Chef's Knife**: A good-quality chef's knife is essential for chopping, slicing, and dicing fruits, vegetables, and other ingredients quickly and efficiently.

**Cutting Board**: Use a durable cutting board to protect your countertops and provide a stable surface for chopping and preparing ingredients.

**Vegetable Peeler**: A vegetable peeler makes it easy to peel fruits and vegetables, removing the skin and making them ready for consumption or cooking.

**Blender or Food Processor**: A blender or food processor is versatile for making smoothies, soups, sauces, and dips using fruits, vegetables, and other nutritious ingredients.

**Salad Spinner:** A salad spinner helps to wash and dry leafy greens thoroughly, making them ready to use in salads, sandwiches, wraps, and other dishes.

**Steamer Basket:** A steamer basket is useful for steaming vegetables, seafood, and other foods while retaining their nutrients and natural flavors.

**Non-Stick Skillet or Pan:** A non-stick skillet or pan is handy for cooking lean proteins, sautéing vegetables, and preparing eggs with minimal added oil or fat.

**Baking Sheet:** A baking sheet is essential for roasting vegetables, baking whole grains, and preparing healthy snacks like roasted chickpeas or kale chips.

**Measuring Cups and Spoons**: Accurately measuring ingredients is crucial for following recipes and portion control, so having a set of measuring cups and spoons is essential.

**Kitchen Scale**: A kitchen scale is helpful for measuring ingredients by weight, especially for precise measurements of grains, proteins, and other foods.

**Mixing Bowls**: Use mixing bowls for combining ingredients, marinating proteins, tossing salads, and preparing dressings and sauces.

**Grater or Zester**: A grater or zester is useful for grating cheese, citrus zest, and other ingredients to add flavor and texture to dishes.

**Strainer or Colander**: A strainer or colander is necessary for draining and rinsing canned beans, vegetables, and grains, as well as washing fruits and vegetables.

**Storage Containers**: Invest in a variety of storage containers for storing leftovers, prepped ingredients, and homemade meals in the refrigerator or freezer.

**Water Bottle**: Staying hydrated is essential for overall health, so having a reusable water bottle on hand encourages regular water intake throughout the day.

**Slow Cooker or Instant Pot**: A slow cooker or Instant Pot is convenient for preparing nutritious meals with minimal effort, such as soups, stews, and one-pot dishes.

# CHAPTER FOUR

## DASH Diet Meal Planning

To make sure you are getting all the nutrients you need, it's critical to balance the different food groups in your meal plans when following the DASH diet. Here are some pointers for DASH diet meal planning:

**Set Your Goals**: Before you start meal planning, identify your health goals and dietary needs. Whether you're looking to lower your blood pressure, manage your weight, or improve overall health, understanding your goals will help you tailor your meal plan accordingly.

**Learn about the DASH Diet**: Become familiar with the main tenets of the DASH diet, which include consuming less salt, saturated fat, and added sugars and more fruits, vegetables, whole grains, lean proteins, and low-fat dairy products.

**Make a Weekly Menu:** Make a weekly meal plan that includes breakfast, lunch, dinner, and snacks. To make sure you're getting enough nutrition, try to eat a balance of foods from each food group that are high in nutrients.

**Incorporate Variety**: Include a variety of foods in your meals to ensure you're getting a wide range of nutrients. Experiment with different fruits, vegetables, whole grains, lean proteins, and healthy fats to keep your meals interesting and satisfying.

**Use Seasonal Ingredients:** Take advantage of seasonal produce to add freshness and flavor to your meals. Seasonal fruits and vegetables are often more affordable and taste better, making them a great choice for DASH diet meal planning.

**Plan for Balanced Meals:** Each meal should include a balance of carbohydrates, protein, and healthy fats, along with plenty of fruits and vegetables. Aim for colorful, nutrient-dense meals that provide sustained energy and keep you feeling full and satisfied.

**Prep Ahead**: Take time to prep ingredients in advance to streamline meal preparation throughout the week. Wash and chop fruits and vegetables, cook grains and beans, and portion out ingredients for easy assembly when it's time to cook.

**Include Snacks**: Plan for healthy snacks to keep you satisfied between meals and prevent unhealthy cravings. Choose options like fresh fruit, cut-up vegetables with hummus, Greek yogurt, nuts, or whole grain crackers with cheese.

**Be Mindful of Portions**: Pay attention to portion sizes to ensure you're not overeating, especially calorie-dense foods like nuts, seeds, and oils. Use measuring cups, spoons, and kitchen scales to help you portion out servings accurately.

**Stay Flexible**: While it's important to have a meal plan, it's also essential to stay flexible and adaptable. Life can be unpredictable, so be prepared to make adjustments to your meal plan based on changes in schedule, preferences, or availability of ingredients.

**Monitor Sodium Intake**: Be mindful of sodium content when planning meals and choose lower-sodium options whenever possible. Use herbs, spices, and other flavorings to enhance the taste of your dishes without relying on salt.

**Track Your Progress**: Keep track of your meals and snacks to monitor your progress and identify areas for improvement. This can help you stay accountable and make adjustments to your meal plan as needed.

# Planning Balanced Meals

Here are some pointers for organizing healthy meals while following the DASH diet:

**Put an Emphasis on Fruits and Vegetables**: Try to incorporate a range of fruits and veggies into each meal. They include a lot of antioxidants, vitamins, and minerals.
Add colorful veggies like bell peppers, carrots, and tomatoes, along with leafy greens like spinach, kale, and Swiss chard.

**Choose Whole Grains:**
Opt for whole grains such as brown rice, quinoa, barley, oats, whole wheat bread, and whole grain pasta.
Whole grains are high in fiber, which helps promote heart health and maintain stable blood sugar levels.

**Include Lean Proteins:**
Choose lean sources of protein such as
skinless poultry, fish, tofu, tempeh, legumes
(beans, lentils, chickpeas), and low-fat dairy
products.
Limit red meat consumption and choose lean
cuts when you do eat it.

**Incorporate Dairy:**
Select low-fat or non-fat dairy products like
milk, yogurt, and cheese.
Dairy products are excellent sources of calcium
and protein, important for bone health and
muscle function.

**Limit Sodium**: Instead of using salt to flavor
food, try utilizing herbs, spices, and lemon juice
to lower your sodium intake.
Steer clear of packaged and processed foods
because they frequently have high salt content.

**Incorporate Good Fats:** Pick foods like avocados, almonds, seeds, and olive oil that are rich in good fats.
When ingested in moderation, these fats promote heart health and help lower inflammation.

**Sample Day Meal Plan:**

**Breakfast**:
Whole grain oatmeal topped with sliced strawberries and a handful of walnuts.
A side of Greek yogurt with honey and a sprinkle of chia seeds.
A glass of freshly squeezed orange juice.

**Snack:**
Sliced cucumber and carrot sticks with hummus.

**Lunch:**
salad of grilled chicken breasts, cucumbers,
cherry tomatoes, and mixed greens dressed
with a balsamic vinaigrette.
a roll made entirely of grains.
a fresh fruit slice, like an apple or a pear.

**Snack**:
Low-fat cottage cheese with pineapple chunks.

**Dinner:**
Baked salmon seasoned with herbs and
lemon.
Quinoa pilaf with sautéed spinach, bell
peppers, and onions.
Steamed broccoli drizzled with olive oil.
A mixed berry parfait for dessert, made with
Greek yogurt and topped with a sprinkle of
granola.

**Tips**:
To make sure you have all the ingredients on hand, plan your meals in advance.
To keep meals tasty and interesting, try experimenting with different recipes and cooking techniques.
Drink lots of water throughout the day to stay hydrated.
Even with nutritious foods, watch your portion amounts to prevent overindulging.
Because maintaining a healthy weight is crucial for heart health, pay attention to how many calories you consume overall.

# Weekly Meal Planning Guide

This weekly meal planning tool will assist you in adhering to the Dash Diet:

**Day 1:**

**Breakfast:**
sliced tomatoes and mashed avocado on top of whole grain bread.
Eggs scrambled with spinach.
slices of fresh oranges.

**Lunch**:
Quinoa salad with diced cucumbers, cherry tomatoes, black beans, corn, and a lime-cilantro dressing.
A side of Greek yogurt with a drizzle of honey.

**Dinner:**
Baked salmon with a lemon-dill sauce.
Steamed green beans.
Brown rice pilaf with diced carrots and peas.

**Day 2:**

**Breakfast**
Almond milk, chia seeds, mixed berries, and
rolled oats are the ingredients for overnight
oats.
A few almonds in a handful.

**Lunch:**
Grilled chicken breast salad with mixed greens,
bell peppers, cucumbers, and a light vinaigrette
dressing.
Whole grain roll.

**Dinner**:
Lentil and vegetable stew served with a side of
whole grain bread.
Steamed broccoli.

**Day 3:**

**Breakfast:**
Greek yogurt parfait with layers of yogurt,
granola, and fresh fruit (such as strawberries
and blueberries).

**Lunch**:
Whole wheat wrap filled with hummus, sliced
turkey breast, lettuce, tomatoes, and
cucumbers.
Baby carrots on the side.

**Dinner:**
Marinara sauce and whole wheat spaghetti are
served with turkey meatballs.
asparagus cooked in steam.

**Day 4:**

**Breakfast:**
Whole grain waffles topped with sliced
bananas and a drizzle of maple syrup.
A glass of skim milk.

**Lunch:**
Quinoa and black bean stuffed bell peppers.
Mixed green salad with a balsamic vinaigrette.

**Dinner:**
Brown rice with stir-fried tofu, broccoli, bell peppers, and snap peas.
Dessert is slices of orange.

**Day 5:**

**Breakfast:**
spinach, tomatoes, mushrooms, and egg whites are used to make a vegetarian omelet.
toast with whole grains.

**Lunch:**
Lentil soup with a side of whole grain crackers.
A small apple.

**Dinner:**
Grilled shrimp skewers with a side of quinoa salad (quinoa mixed with diced cucumber, cherry tomatoes, feta cheese, and lemon vinaigrette).
Steamed Brussels sprouts.

**Day 6:**

**Breakfast:**
Smoothie made with spinach, kale, banana,
frozen berries, and almond milk.
A handful of walnuts.

**Lunch**
A whole wheat tortilla topped with a turkey and
avocado wrap along with lettuce, tomato, and
mustard.
Hummus on sticks with carrots.

**Dinner**
roasted sweet potatoes and green beans
paired with baked chicken breast.
a cucumber, mixed greens, and light dressing
side salad.

**Day 7:**

**Breakfast:**
Whole grain English muffin topped with almond
butter and sliced strawberries.
A glass of orange juice.

**Lunch:**
Quinoa and chickpea salad with diced bell
peppers, cucumbers, and a lemon-tahini
dressing.
Greek yogurt is reduced in fat and drizzled with
honey.

**Dinner:**
Grilled vegetable skewers (zucchini, bell
peppers, onions) served with whole wheat
couscous.
Mixed berry salad for dessert (berries topped
with a dollop of Greek yogurt).

**Tips for Weekly Meal Planning:**
Make a shopping list based on your meal plan
to ensure you have all the necessary
ingredients.
To save time during the week, prepare
ingredients ahead of time, such as chopping
vegetables or cooking grains.
Be adaptable with your food plan, modifying it
as necessary to fit your preferences and
timetable.
Think about cooking some foods in bulk, such
as grains or proteins, so you can utilize them in
several meals a week.
To make sure you're getting a variety of
nutrients, try to vary up your meals.

# Sample Meal Plans

**Breakfast**:
oatmeal with almond strews and fresh berries
on top.
Greek yogurt on the side, drizzled with honey.
A fresh fruit piece or a glass of orange juice.

**Mid-Morning Snack:**
A small handful of unsalted nuts (like almonds
or walnuts).
Sliced vegetables (such as carrots or
cucumbers) with hummus.

**Lunch:**
Grilled chicken breast served with a mixed
green salad (spinach, kale, arugula) topped
with cherry tomatoes, cucumbers, and a
vinaigrette dressing.
A side of quinoa or brown rice.
A piece of fruit for dessert, like an apple or a
pear.

**Afternoon Snack:**
Low-fat cottage cheese with sliced peaches or
pineapple.
Whole grain crackers with a small amount of
natural peanut butter.

**Dinner:**
Baked salmon seasoned with herbs and
lemon.
Steamed broccoli and carrots.
A small serving of whole wheat pasta with
marinara sauce.
A mixed green salad with balsamic vinaigrette.
A slice of whole grain bread.
Evening Snack:
A small bowl of mixed berries.
A glass of low-fat milk or a cup of herbal tea.

**Fluids:**
Make it a point to stay hydrated during the day.
Limit alcohol and sugar-filled beverage
consumption.

**Additional Tips:**
Choose whole grains over refined grains.
Option for lean protein sources like poultry,
fish, beans, and legumes.
At every meal, include an ample amount of
fruits and vegetables.
Instead of using salt to flavor meals, use herbs
and spices.
Cut back on packaged and processed foods,
which are frequently heavy in fat and sodium.

Remember to adjust portion sizes according to
your individual calorie and nutrient needs, and
consult with a healthcare professional or a
registered dietitian before making significant
changes to your diet, especially if you have any
underlying health conditions.

# CHAPTER FIVE

## Delicious DASH Diet Recipes

Delicious DASH diet recipes offer flavorful and nutritious options that adhere to the principles of the Dietary Approaches to Stop Hypertension (DASH) diet. These recipes focus on incorporating nutrient-rich ingredients such as fruits, vegetables, whole grains, lean proteins, and healthy fats while minimizing sodium, saturated fats, and cholesterol. Here's a comprehensive overview of some popular DASH diet recipes:

**Salads and Bowls:**
Colorful salads bursting with fresh vegetables, fruits, and leafy greens provide a variety of vitamins, minerals, and antioxidants.
Grain bowls featuring whole grains like quinoa or brown rice, paired with lean proteins such as

grilled chicken or tofu, and topped with an assortment of veggies and a flavorful dressing. Bean salads combine fiber-rich beans like chickpeas, black beans, or kidney beans with chopped vegetables, herbs, and a tangy vinaigrette.

**Soups and Stews:**
Vegetable-packed soups and stews simmered with herbs and spices offer a comforting and satisfying meal option.
Lentil soup or chili made with protein-rich lentils, tomatoes, carrots, celery, and onions, seasoned with garlic, cumin, and paprika for added flavor.
Minestrone soup is loaded with a variety of colorful vegetables like zucchini, bell peppers, and spinach, along with whole wheat pasta and white beans.

**Grilled and Baked Dishes:**
Grilled or baked fish seasoned with herbs, lemon, and a touch of olive oil provides heart-healthy omega-3 fatty acids and lean protein.

Marinated chicken or tofu skewers cooked on the grill or in the oven with a flavorful marinade made from herbs, garlic, and citrus juices. Roasted vegetables such as sweet potatoes, Brussels sprouts, and cauliflower tossed with olive oil and herbs, then roasted until caramelized and tender.

**Whole Grain Delights:**
Whole grain pasta dishes featuring whole wheat or brown rice pasta tossed with a variety of vegetables, lean proteins, and a light tomato or pesto sauce.
Whole grain breakfast options like oatmeal topped with fresh berries, nuts, and a drizzle of honey, or whole grain pancakes served with Greek yogurt and sliced fruit.
Whole grain wraps or sandwiches filled with lean meats, hummus, avocado, and plenty of veggies for a satisfying and nutritious meal.

**Snacks and Treats:**
Nutrient-packed snacks such as sliced vegetables with hummus, Greek yogurt with fruit and a sprinkle of nuts, or whole grain crackers with cheese provide satisfying options between meals.
Fruit smoothies made with fresh or frozen fruits, Greek yogurt, and a splash of milk or juice offer a refreshing and nutritious treat. Homemade trail mix combining unsalted nuts, seeds, dried fruits, and a sprinkle of dark chocolate chips for a satisfying and portable snack.

**Stuffed Bell Peppers:** Fill bell peppers with a mixture of cooked quinoa, lean ground turkey or tofu, black beans, corn, diced tomatoes, and spices like cumin and chili powder. After the filling is thoroughly heated and the peppers are soft, bake them.

**Mediterranean Chickpea Salad**: Combine cooked chickpeas with diced cucumbers, cherry tomatoes, red onion, Kalamata olives, and crumbled feta cheese. Dress with a mixture of olive oil, lemon juice, minced garlic, and oregano for a refreshing and satisfying salad.

**Vegetable and Lentil Soup:** In a large pot, sauté diced onions, carrots, celery, and garlic in olive oil until softened. Add low-sodium vegetable broth, dried lentils, diced tomatoes, and a variety of chopped vegetables such as spinach, kale, and bell peppers. Simmer until lentils are tender and flavors are well blended.

# Breakfasts

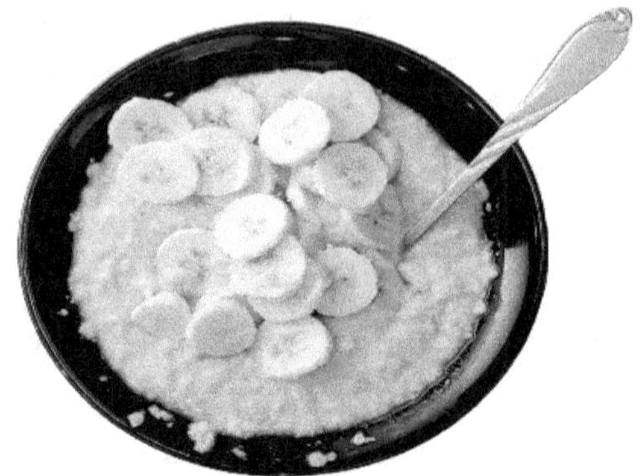

## DASH Diet Oatmeal Bowl:

A DASH diet oatmeal bowl is a nutritious and satisfying breakfast option that aligns with the principles of the Dietary Approaches to Stop Hypertension (DASH) diet. Here's how to make one and its health benefits:

**Recipe for DASH Diet Oatmeal Bowl:**

**Ingredients:**
1/2 cup old-fashioned oats
1 cup water or low-fat milk (such as almond or
skim milk)
Fresh fruit (e.g., sliced bananas, berries, diced
apples)
Nuts or seeds, such as chia seeds, walnuts,
and almonds
Greek yogurt, honey, and cinnamon are
optional toppings.

**Instructions:**
Heat the milk or water in a saucepan until it
begins to boil.
After adding the oats, turn down the heat.
Cook, stirring periodically, until liquid thickens
to desired consistency and oats are cooked, 5
to 7 minutes.
Take it off the stove and give it a minute to rest.
After cooking, transfer the oatmeal to a bowl.

Add any extra desired toppings, such as nuts
or seeds, and fresh fruit on top.
If desired, sprinkle with cinnamon or drizzle
with honey.
Enjoy it while it's hot!

**Health Benefits of DASH Diet Oatmeal
Bowl:**

**Heart Health**: Oats are rich in soluble fiber,
which can help lower LDL (bad) cholesterol
levels, reducing the risk of heart disease. The
DASH diet emphasizes foods like oats that
promote heart health.

**Blood Pressure Regulation**: The DASH diet
is specifically designed to lower blood
pressure, and oatmeal fits well into this plan.
Oats contain beta-glucans, a type of soluble
fiber that has been shown to help regulate
blood pressure.

**Weight Management**: Oatmeal is a filling breakfast option that can help keep you satisfied until your next meal. The fiber in oats slows digestion, prolonging feelings of fullness and reducing the likelihood of overeating later in the day.

**Nutrient Density**: Adding fresh fruit to your oatmeal bowl increases its nutrient content, providing essential vitamins, minerals, and antioxidants. Nuts and seeds contribute healthy fats, protein, and additional fiber, further enhancing the nutritional profile of the meal.

**Consistent Energy Release**: The complex carbs in oatmeal allow the body to break them down gradually, giving you a constant boost of energy throughout the morning. This can help you stay focused and awake by preventing energy crashes.

# Veggie Omelet with Feta

A Veggie Omelet with Feta is a nutritious and flavorful breakfast option that aligns perfectly with the principles of the DASH (Dietary Approaches to Stop Hypertension) diet. Here's a comprehensive explanation of how to make it and its health benefits:

**Recipe for Veggie Omelet with Feta:**

**Ingredients**:
2 large eggs
1/4 cup diced bell peppers (any color)
1/4 cup diced tomatoes
1/4 cup chopped spinach
2 tablespoons crumbled feta cheese
1 teaspoon olive oil
Salt and pepper to taste
Fresh herbs (optional for garnish).

**Instructions:**
In a nonstick skillet, warm the olive oil over medium heat.
Cook the chopped bell peppers for two to three

minutes, or until they start to soften.

Cook the chopped spinach and diced tomatoes in the skillet for a further one to two minutes, or until the spinach wilts.

Whisk the eggs with the salt and pepper in a small bowl.

Evenly cover the vegetables in the skillet with the egg mixture.

Cook for 2-3 minutes, lifting the edges of the omelet with a spatula to let the uncooked egg flow underneath.

Once the omelet is mostly set but still slightly runny on top, sprinkle the crumbled feta cheese evenly over one half of the omelet.

Using a spatula, carefully fold the other half of the omelet over the cheese to create a half-moon shape.

Cook for another 1-2 minutes until the cheese melts and the omelet is cooked through.

Slide the omelet onto a plate, garnish with fresh herbs if desired, and serve hot.

**Health Benefits of Veggie Omelet with Feta for DASH Diet:**

**High in Protein:** Eggs are a rich source of high-quality protein, which is essential for muscle repair, maintenance, and overall health. Including protein in your breakfast helps keep you feeling full and satisfied until your next meal, promoting weight management and stable energy levels.

**Packed with Vegetables**: This omelet is loaded with nutrient-rich vegetables like bell peppers, tomatoes, and spinach. Vegetables are low in calories but high in vitamins, minerals, and antioxidants, which support overall health and reduce the risk of chronic diseases such as heart disease and cancer.

**Rich in Healthy Fats**: Olive oil and feta cheese provide healthy fats, including monounsaturated fats and omega-3 fatty acids, which have been shown to reduce inflammation, lower cholesterol levels, and improve heart health. Consuming moderate amounts of healthy fats is an important aspect of the DASH diet.

**Low in Sodium:** Feta cheese adds a burst of flavor to the omelet without the need for extra salt. Reducing sodium intake is a key component of the DASH diet, as excessive sodium consumption can contribute to high blood pressure and other cardiovascular issues.

**Versatile and Customizable**: This recipe is highly adaptable to personal preferences and dietary restrictions. You can easily customize the omelet by adding or omitting vegetables, adjusting the amount of cheese, or incorporating fresh herbs and spices for added flavor without extra calories or sodium.

# Banana Walnut Pancakes

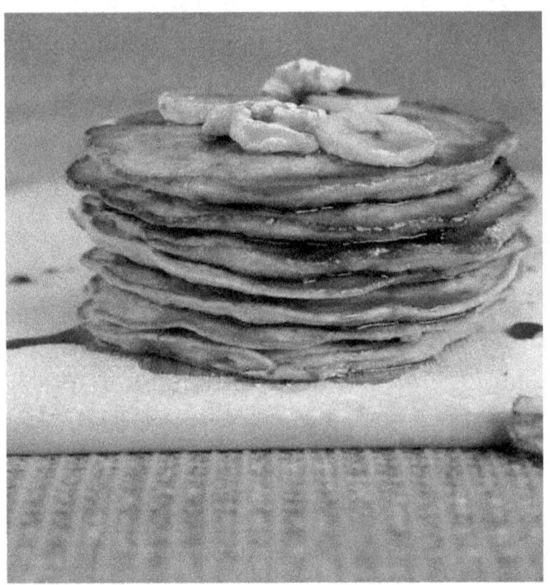

Banana walnut pancakes are a delicious and nutritious breakfast option that can be adapted to fit the Dietary Approaches to Stop Hypertension (DASH) diet. Here's a comprehensive explanation:

**Ingredients:**

**Whole wheat flour**: Provides fiber and nutrients compared to refined white flour.
Ripe bananas: Adds natural sweetness, potassium, and fiber.
**Chopped walnuts**: Rich in omega-3 fatty acids, protein, and antioxidants.
**Eggs:** A good source of protein and essential nutrients.
Milk (preferably low-fat or non-dairy alternatives like almond milk): Adds moisture and protein.

**Baking powder:** Helps the pancakes rise.
Cinnamon and vanilla extract: Adds flavor without extra calories.
A tiny bit of honey or maple syrup, if preferred, is optional.

**Preparation**:
Mash the ripe bananas in a mixing bowl.
Add eggs, milk, vanilla extract, and any optional sweeteners, then whisk until well combined.

In a separate bowl, mix together the whole wheat flour, baking powder, cinnamon, and chopped walnuts.
Gradually add the dry ingredients to the wet ingredients, stirring until just combined. Be careful not to overmix.
Heat a non-stick skillet or griddle over medium heat and lightly coat with cooking spray or a small amount of oil.
Pour a portion of the pancake batter onto the skillet, using about 1/4 cup for each pancake.

Fry until surface bubbles appear, then turn and continue cooking until both sides are golden brown.
If preferred, top warm servings with chopped walnuts, more banana slices, and a honey or maple syrup drizzle.

## Health Benefits

**Rich in Fiber:** Whole wheat flour and bananas provide dietary fiber, which promotes digestive health and helps regulate blood sugar levels.

**Heart-Healthy Fats:** Walnuts are a great source of omega-3 fatty acids, which can help reduce inflammation and lower the risk of heart disease.

**Potassium:** Bananas are high in potassium, a mineral that plays a crucial role in maintaining healthy blood pressure levels, making this recipe ideal for the DASH diet, which emphasizes potassium-rich foods.

**Low in Added Sugar**: By using ripe bananas for sweetness and minimal added sweeteners, this recipe keeps added sugar levels low, which aligns with the DASH diet's focus on reducing sugar intake.

**Balanced Nutrients**: The combination of whole wheat flour, eggs, and milk provides a balance of carbohydrates, protein, and essential vitamins and minerals, making these pancakes a nutritious and satisfying breakfast option for those following the DASH diet.

# Greek Yogurt Parfait

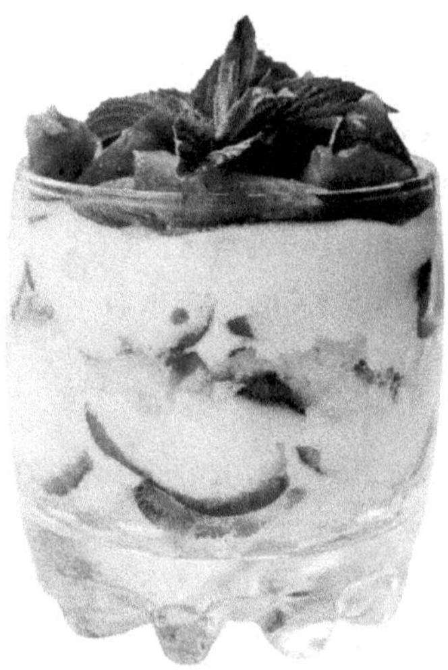

A Greek yogurt parfait is a nutritious and delicious breakfast or snack option that fits well within the guidelines of the Dietary Approaches to Stop Hypertension (DASH) diet. Here's a comprehensive explanation:

**Ingredients:**

**Greek yogurt**: Provides protein, probiotics for gut health, and calcium.
Fresh fruits **(such as berries, sliced bananas, or diced mango):** Adds natural sweetness, vitamins, minerals, and fiber.
**Whole grain granola or oats:** Adds crunch, fiber, and additional nutrients.
**Optional**: nuts (such as almonds, walnuts, or pecans) or seeds (such as chia seeds or flaxseeds) for added texture and healthy fats.
Optional: a drizzle of honey or maple syrup for sweetness (if desired).

**Preparation**:
Start by layering a few spoonfuls of Greek yogurt into a glass or bowl.
Add a layer of fresh fruits on top of the yogurt.
Sprinkle a layer of granola or oats over the fruit.

Once the glass or bowl is full, continue layering until a final layer of yogurt is on top.
Optionally, drizzle honey or maple syrup over the top for added sweetness.
Garnish with nuts or seeds for extra texture and nutrition.

**Health Benefits for the DASH Diet:**

**High in Protein**: Greek yogurt is a rich source of protein, which helps promote satiety, stabilize blood sugar levels, and support muscle health.

**Probiotics:** Greek yogurt contains probiotics, beneficial bacteria that promote gut health and may improve digestion and immune function.

**Calcium:** Greek yogurt is also a good source of calcium, essential for maintaining strong bones and teeth.

**Fiber**: Adding fresh fruits and whole grain granola or oats to the parfait increases its fiber content, which supports digestive health and helps regulate blood sugar levels.

**Heart-Healthy Fats:** Nuts and seeds are excellent sources of heart-healthy fats, such as omega-3 fatty acids, which can help reduce inflammation and lower the risk of heart disease.

**Low in Added Sugar**: By using fresh fruits for sweetness and minimal added sweeteners, this recipe keeps added sugar levels low, aligning with the DASH diet's focus on reducing sugar intake.

**Nutrient Density:** Greek yogurt parfait is packed with essential vitamins, minerals, antioxidants, and other nutrients, making it a nutrient-dense option for those following the DASH diet.

# Lunches

## Mediterranean Chickpea Salad

Mediterranean chickpea salad is a flavorful and nutritious dish inspired by the traditional Mediterranean diet, which has been associated with numerous health benefits, including reduced risk of heart disease and improved overall well-being. This salad aligns well with the principles of the Dietary Approaches to Stop Hypertension (DASH) diet. Here's a comprehensive explanation:

**Ingredients:**

**Chickpeas (also known as garbanzo beans):** High in protein, fiber, and essential nutrients such as folate, iron, and manganese.
**Cucumber**: Adds hydration, crunch, and vitamins such as vitamin K and vitamin C.
**Tomatoes**: Provide antioxidants such as lycopene, as well as vitamins and minerals.
Red onion: Adds flavor and a dose of antioxidants.

**Kalamata olives**: Add a salty tang and healthy monounsaturated fats.

**Fresh parsley**: Adds freshness and nutrients such as vitamin K and vitamin C.

**Feta cheese (optional):** Adds creaminess and a hint of tanginess.

Antioxidants and heart-healthy monounsaturated fats are included in extra virgin olive oil.

**Lemon juice**: Adds acidity and brightness.

**Garlic:** Adds flavor and potential health benefits, including immune support.

Salt and pepper: To taste.


**Preparation**:

Rinse and drain the chickpeas if using canned food.

Chop the cucumber, tomatoes, red onion, and parsley.

In a large bowl, combine the chickpeas, chopped vegetables, and olives.

To create the dressing, combine the lemon juice, extra virgin olive oil, minced garlic, salt, and pepper in a small bowl.

After adding the dressing to the salad, stir to fully incorporate.
If using, crumble the feta cheese on top of the salad.
Serve immediately or chill in the refrigerator for a couple of hours to allow the flavors to meld.

**Health Benefits for the DASH Diet:**

**High in Fiber**: Chickpeas and vegetables in the salad are high in fiber, which promotes digestive health, helps control blood sugar levels, and supports weight management.
**Heart-Healthy Fats**: Extra virgin olive oil and olives provide monounsaturated fats, which can help reduce LDL (bad) cholesterol levels and lower the risk of heart disease.

**Low in Sodium**: By using minimal added salt and incorporating flavorful ingredients like olives and lemon juice, this salad can be low in sodium, which is important for managing blood pressure as recommended by the DASH diet.

**Rich in Antioxidants**: Tomatoes, parsley, garlic, and olives are rich in antioxidants, which help protect cells from damage caused by free radicals and may reduce the risk of chronic diseases.

**Potassium:** Chickpeas and vegetables are good sources of potassium, an essential mineral that helps regulate blood pressure and counteract the effects of sodium in the body.

**Versatile and Nutrient-Dense:** This salad is highly customizable and can be adapted to include other Mediterranean-inspired ingredients like bell peppers, artichoke hearts, or spinach, while still providing a variety of essential nutrients and flavors.

Overall, Mediterranean chickpea salad is a delicious and satisfying option for a DASH diet meal plan, offering a balance of protein, fiber, healthy fats, vitamins, minerals, and antioxidants to support heart health, blood pressure management, and overall well-being.

# Turkey and Avocado Wrap

A Turkey and Avocado Wrap is a delicious and nutritious meal option that aligns well with the principles of the Dietary Approaches to Stop Hypertension (DASH) diet. Here's a comprehensive explanation:

**Ingredients:**

**Whole grain or whole wheat tortilla:** Provides fiber, vitamins, and minerals compared to refined white tortillas.
**Sliced turkey breast**: Offers lean protein, which supports muscle health and helps keep you feeling full and satisfied.
**Ripe avocado:** Adds healthy fats, fiber, vitamins (such as vitamin K, vitamin C, vitamin E, and B-vitamins), minerals (including potassium, magnesium, and folate), and antioxidants.
**Leafy greens (such as lettuce or spinach):** Adds texture, flavor, and additional vitamins and minerals.

**Sliced tomatoes:** Provides hydration, vitamins (including vitamin C), minerals, and antioxidants.

**Optional:** mustard or hummus for added flavor and moisture.

**Optional:** red onion, sprouts, shredded carrots, or cucumber slices for extra crunch and nutrients.

**Preparation:**

Lay the whole grain tortilla flat on a clean surface.

Layer the sliced turkey breast, avocado slices, leafy greens, and sliced tomatoes evenly over the tortilla.

If desired, spread a thin layer of mustard or hummus over the ingredients for added flavor and moisture.

Add any optional toppings, such as red onion, sprouts, shredded carrots, or cucumber slices.

To construct a wrap, carefully roll up the tortilla, tucking in the edges as you go.

If desired, cut the wrap in half diagonally to make eating simpler.
Serve right away or store carefully wrapped in foil or parchment paper for later use.

**Health Benefits for the DASH Diet:**

**Lean Protein**: Turkey breast is a lean source of protein, which helps build and repair tissues, support immune function, and maintain muscle mass. Choosing lean proteins like turkey aligns with the DASH diet's emphasis on reducing saturated fat intake.

**Healthy Fats**: Avocado provides heart-healthy monounsaturated fats, which can help lower LDL (bad) cholesterol levels and reduce the risk of heart disease. The combination of lean protein from turkey and healthy fats from avocado makes this wrap a balanced and satisfying meal option.

**Fiber**: Whole grain tortillas, avocado, and vegetables in the wrap are rich in fiber, which supports digestive health, helps control blood sugar levels, and promotes satiety. Adequate fiber intake is an important component of the DASH diet.

**Vitamins and Minerals:** Avocado, leafy greens, and tomatoes are packed with essential vitamins (such as vitamin C, vitamin K, and vitamin E) and minerals (including potassium, magnesium, and folate), which contribute to overall health and well-being.

**Low in Sodium**: By using minimally processed ingredients and controlling added salt, this turkey and avocado wrap can be a low-sodium option suitable for those following the DASH diet, which emphasizes reducing sodium intake to help manage blood pressure.

**Versatile and Convenient**: This wrap is highly customizable and can be adapted to include a variety of vegetables, herbs, or condiments while still providing a nutritious and satisfying meal option for those following the DASH diet.

# Quinoa Stuffed Bell Peppers

Quinoa stuffed bell peppers are a nutritious and flavorful dish that fits well within the Dietary Approaches to Stop Hypertension (DASH) diet guidelines. Here's a comprehensive explanation:

**Ingredients:**

**Bell peppers**: Rich in vitamins A and C, fiber, and antioxidants.
**Quinoa:** A complete protein source containing all nine essential amino acids, fiber, vitamins, and minerals such as magnesium and iron.
Lean ground turkey or chicken (optional): Adds protein and flavor.
**Onion:** Adds flavor and nutrients such as vitamin C and fiber.
**Garlic:** Enhances flavor and offers potential health benefits, including immune support.
**Tomatoes**: Provide lycopene, vitamins, and minerals.

**Spinach or kale**: Adds fiber, vitamins (such as vitamin K), minerals, and antioxidants.
Low-sodium vegetable or chicken broth: Adds moisture and flavor.
Herbs and spices (such as parsley, basil, **oregano, and paprika):** Enhance flavor without extra calories.
Optional: Feta cheese or grated Parmesan cheese for topping.

**Preparation:**
Preheat the oven to 375°F (190°C).
Slice off the bell peppers' tops, then take out the seeds and membranes. The peppers should be put on a baking tray.
Cook the quinoa according to package instructions.
In a skillet, cook the ground turkey or chicken (if using) until browned. Add chopped onion and garlic and cook until softened.
Stir in diced tomatoes and chopped spinach or kale, and cook until wilted.
Stir thoroughly after adding the cooked quinoa to the skillet. To taste, add more spices and herbs for flavor.

Fill the hollowed-out bell peppers halfway with the quinoa mixture, packing it down.
Fill the baking dish's bottom with the vegetable or chicken broth.
Once the peppers are soft, bake the baking dish covered with foil for 25 to 30 minutes.
For the final five minutes of baking, top the filled peppers with cheese, if using.
Enjoy it while it's hot!

**Health Benefits for the DASH Diet:**

**High in Fiber:** Quinoa, bell peppers, and leafy greens are rich in fiber, which supports digestive health, helps control blood sugar levels, and promotes satiety.

**Lean Protein:** Lean ground turkey or chicken provides protein, which is essential for muscle health, immune function, and satiety. This lean protein option aligns with the DASH diet's recommendation to reduce saturated fat intake.

**Low in Sodium**: By using low-sodium vegetable or chicken broth and controlling added salt, this recipe can be low in sodium, which is important for managing blood pressure as recommended by the DASH diet.

**Heart-Healthy Ingredients**: Bell peppers, tomatoes, spinach or kale, and herbs and spices are all rich in vitamins, minerals, and antioxidants that support heart health and overall well-being.

**Nutrient Density**: Quinoa stuffed bell peppers are packed with essential nutrients, including protein, fiber, vitamins (such as vitamin A, vitamin C, and vitamin K), minerals (such as magnesium, iron, and potassium), and antioxidants, making them a nutrient-dense option for those following the DASH diet.

**Versatility**: This recipe is highly customizable and can be adapted to include other vegetables, herbs, or spices while still providing a nutritious and satisfying meal option for those following the DASH diet.

# Dinners

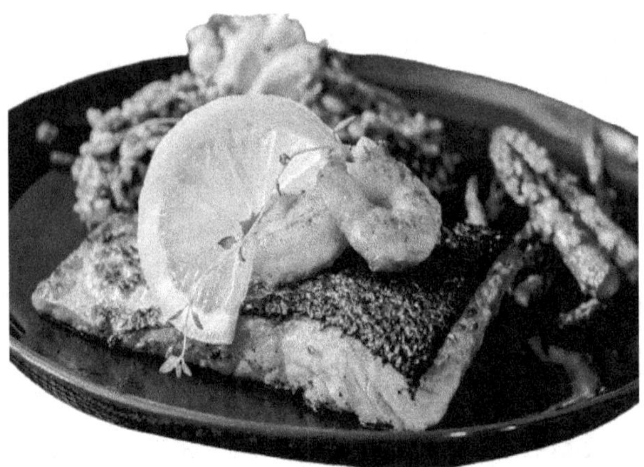

## Grilled Salmon with Asparagus

A tasty and healthy dish that fits in nicely with the DASH (Dietary Approaches to Stop Hypertension) diet's tenets is grilled salmon with asparagus. This is a thorough explanation:

**Ingredients:**

**Salmon filets:** A rich source of omega-3 fatty acids, high-quality protein, and essential nutrients such as vitamin D, vitamin B12, and selenium.

**Fresh asparagus spears**: Provide fiber, vitamins (such as vitamin A, vitamin C, and vitamin K), minerals (including folate and potassium), and antioxidants.
**Olive oil:** Rich in antioxidants and heart-healthy monounsaturated fats.
Lemon juice: Adds acidity and brightness to the dish.
**Garlic**: Enhances flavor and offers potential health benefits, including immune support.

**Herbs and spices (such as dill, parsley, thyme, or black pepper):** Enhance flavor without extra calories.
**Optional:** sea salt or low-sodium seasoning blend for added flavor (if desired).

**Preparation:**
Preheat the grill to medium-high heat.
In a small bowl, mix together olive oil, lemon juice, minced garlic, herbs, and spices to make the marinade.

Place the salmon filets and asparagus spears
in separate shallow dishes or resealable plastic
bags.
Pour the marinade over the salmon filets and
asparagus spears, ensuring they are evenly
coated.
Give them 15 to 30 minutes to marinade.
Remove the salmon filets and asparagus
spears from the marinade, shaking off any
excess.
Grill the salmon filets skin-side down for about
4-5 minutes per side, or until cooked through
and flaky. Grill the asparagus spears for about
3-5 minutes, turning occasionally, until tender
and lightly charred.
Remove the grilled salmon and asparagus
from the grill and serve immediately.
Before serving, you might want to add some
fresh herbs and a squeeze of lemon juice.
asparagus from the grill and serve immediately.
Optionally, garnish with fresh herbs and a
squeeze of lemon juice before serving.

**Health Benefits for the DASH Diet:**

**Omega-3 Fatty Acids**: Salmon is rich in omega-3 fatty acids, particularly EPA and DHA, which have been shown to reduce inflammation, lower triglyceride levels, and support heart health. Consuming omega-3 fatty acids aligns with the DASH diet's emphasis on reducing the risk of heart disease.

**Lean Protein**: Salmon provides high-quality protein, which is essential for muscle health, satiety, and overall well-being. Choosing lean protein sources like salmon aligns with the DASH diet's recommendation to limit saturated fat intake.

**Fiber**: Asparagus is a good source of dietary fiber, which supports digestive health, helps control blood sugar levels, and promotes satiety. Adequate fiber intake is an important component of the DASH diet.

**Vitamins and Minerals:** Salmon and asparagus are both packed with essential vitamins (such as vitamin A, vitamin C, vitamin K, and various B-vitamins) and minerals (including potassium, magnesium, and folate), which contribute to overall health and well-being.

**Antioxidants**: Both salmon and asparagus contain antioxidants, which help protect cells from damage caused by free radicals and may reduce the risk of chronic diseases.

**Heart-Healthy Fats:** Olive oil used in the marinade provides heart-healthy monounsaturated fats, which can help lower LDL (bad) cholesterol levels and reduce the risk of heart disease.

**Low in Sodium**: By using minimal added salt and controlling the use of seasoning blends, this recipe can be low in sodium, which is important for managing blood pressure as recommended by the DASH diet.

# Chicken and Vegetable Stir-Fry

Stir-fried chicken and vegetables is a healthy and adaptable recipe that fits in nicely with the DASH (Dietary Approaches to Stop Hypertension) dietary guidelines. This is a thorough explanation:

**Ingredients:**

Boneless, skinless chicken breast or thigh: Provides lean protein, which supports muscle health and helps keep you feeling full and satisfied.

**Assorted vegetables (such as bell peppers, broccoli, carrots, snap peas, mushrooms, and onions):** Provide fiber, vitamins (such as vitamin A, vitamin C, and vitamin K), minerals (including potassium and magnesium), and antioxidants.

**Low-sodium soy sauce or tamari**: Adds flavor without extra sodium.

**Fresh ginger and garlic**: Enhance flavor and offer potential health benefits, including immune support.

**Olive oil or sesame oil**: Contains heart-healthy monounsaturated fats and adds richness to the dish.
Optional: brown rice, quinoa, or whole grain noodles for serving.

**Preparation:**
Slice the chicken breast or thigh into thin strips and marinate them in a mixture of low-sodium soy sauce or tamari, minced ginger, and minced garlic for about 15-30 minutes.
Prepare the vegetables by washing, peeling (if necessary), and chopping them into bite-sized pieces.
Heat a large skillet or wok over medium-high heat and add a small amount of olive oil or sesame oil.
Add the marinated chicken to the skillet and cook until browned and cooked through, about 5-7 minutes.
After removing it from the skillet, set the chicken aside.

If needed, add a little additional oil to the skillet before adding the chopped veggies. Stir-fry the vegetables for 5 to 7 minutes, or until they are crisp-tender.
Return the cooked chicken to the skillet and toss everything together until well combined and heated through.
Serve the chicken and vegetable stir-fry hot, over cooked brown rice, quinoa, or whole grain noodles if desired.

## Health Benefits for the DASH Diet

**Low in saturated fat:** Chicken and vegetable stir-fry is a lean protein option that is low in saturated fat, making it a heart-healthy choice for those following the DASH diet.

**High in fiber**: Vegetables such as broccoli, bell peppers, and snap peas are high in fiber, which can help promote digestive health and keep you feeling full and satisfied.

**Rich in vitamins and minerals:** This dish is packed with a variety of vitamins and minerals, including vitamin C, vitamin A, and potassium, which are important for overall health and well-being.

**Low in sodium**: By using low-sodium soy sauce and other seasonings, you can control the amount of salt in your stir-fry, making it a suitable option for those looking to reduce their sodium intake as part of the DASH diet.

**Balanced meal**: Chicken provides a good source of protein, while the vegetables offer a variety of nutrients, making this dish a well-rounded and nutritious meal option for those following the DASH diet.

# Lentil Curry with Brown Rice

Lentil curry with brown rice is a flavorful and nutritious dish that aligns well with the principles of the Dietary Approaches to Stop Hypertension (DASH) diet. Here's a comprehensive explanation:

**Ingredients:**

**Lentils:** A good source of plant-based protein, fiber, vitamins (such as folate and vitamin B6), minerals (including iron, potassium, and magnesium), and antioxidants.

**Brown rice**: Provides fiber, vitamins (such as B-vitamins), minerals (including magnesium and selenium), and antioxidants compared to white rice.

**Onion, garlic, and ginger**: Enhance flavor and offer potential health benefits, including immune support.

Assorted vegetables (such as tomatoes, carrots, bell peppers, and spinach): Provide fiber, vitamins (such as vitamin A and vitamin C), minerals, and antioxidants.

**Coconut milk:** Gives the curry taste and creaminess.

Curry powder or curry paste: Provides a blend of spices and herbs, such as turmeric, cumin, coriander, and chili powder, adding flavor and potential health benefits.

**Olive oil or coconut oil:** Contains heart-healthy monounsaturated fats or medium-chain triglycerides (MCTs) and adds richness to the dish.

Optional: fresh cilantro or parsley for garnish.

**Preparation:**

Rinse the lentils and soak them in water for about 30 minutes (optional but can reduce cooking time).

Cook the brown rice according to package instructions.

In a large pot or skillet, heat olive oil or coconut oil over medium heat. Add chopped onion, minced garlic, and grated ginger and cook until softened and fragrant.

Stir in diced tomatoes and chopped vegetables of your choice and cook until they start to soften.

Add drained lentils to the pot along with curry powder or curry paste. Stir to coat the lentils and vegetables with the spices.

Pour in coconut milk and enough water or vegetable broth to cover the lentils and vegetables. After bringing to a simmer, cook for 20 to 30 minutes, or until the lentils are soft.

To taste, add salt and pepper to the lentil curry.

Serve the lentil curry hot over cooked brown rice, garnished with fresh cilantro or parsley if desired.

## Health Benefits for the DASH Diet

**High in fiber**: Lentils and brown rice are both excellent sources of fiber, which can help improve digestion and promote a healthy gut.

**Low in saturated fat**: Lentil curry with brown rice is a heart-healthy meal as it is low in saturated fat, which can help lower cholesterol levels and reduce the risk of heart disease.

**Rich in protein:** Lentils are a great plant-based source of protein, which is essential for muscle growth and repair. Brown rice also contains some protein, making this dish a complete protein source.

**Brimming with micronutrients**: Brown rice is a wonderful source of B vitamins and magnesium, and lentils are high in iron, folate, and potassium. The general health and wellbeing of an individual depends on these nutrients.

**Helps with weight management**: Lentils and brown rice are both low in calories and high in fiber, making them a filling and satisfying meal that can help with weight management.

**Supports blood sugar control:** Lentils and brown rice have a low glycemic index, which means they are digested slowly and can help stabilize blood sugar levels. This can be beneficial for those with diabetes or those looking to manage their blood sugar levels.

# Snacks

## Greek Yogurt with Berries

Greek yogurt with berries is a nutritious and satisfying snack option that aligns well with the principles of the Dietary Approaches to Stop Hypertension (DASH) diet. Here's a comprehensive explanation:

**Ingredients:**

**Greek yogurt**: Provides protein, probiotics for gut health, and calcium.
Fresh berries (such as strawberries, blueberries, raspberries, or blackberries): Adds natural sweetness, vitamins, minerals, and antioxidants.
**Optional**: honey or maple syrup for additional sweetness (if desired).
**Optional**: nuts or seeds (such as almonds, walnuts, chia seeds, or flaxseeds) for added texture and healthy fats.

**Preparation:**
Spoon a serving of Greek yogurt into a bowl or
cup.
Wash the berries and add them on top of the
yogurt.
Drizzle with honey or maple syrup if you prefer
extra sweetness.
Optionally, sprinkle nuts or seeds over the
yogurt and berries for added crunch and
nutrition.
Serve immediately and enjoy!

**Health Benefits for the DASH Diet:**

**High in Protein**: Greek yogurt is a rich source
of protein, which helps promote satiety,
stabilize blood sugar levels, and support
muscle health. Consuming adequate protein
aligns with the DASH diet's emphasis on
nutrient-dense foods that promote fullness and
satisfaction.

**Probiotics**: Greek yogurt contains probiotics, beneficial bacteria that promote gut health and may improve digestion and immune function. A healthy gut microbiome is associated with better overall health and may contribute to lower blood pressure, making Greek yogurt a valuable addition to the DASH diet.

**Calcium**: Greek yogurt is also a good source of calcium, essential for maintaining strong bones and teeth. Adequate calcium intake is important for overall health and may contribute to reduced risk of hypertension.

**Antioxidants**: Berries are packed with antioxidants, including flavonoids and anthocyanins, which help protect cells from damage caused by free radicals and may reduce the risk of chronic diseases such as heart disease and hypertension.

**Fiber:** Berries are also rich in fiber, which supports digestive health, helps control blood sugar levels, and promotes satiety. Consuming fiber-rich foods is a key component of the DASH diet for maintaining overall health and managing blood pressure.

**Heart-Healthy Fats**: Adding nuts or seeds to Greek yogurt and berries provides heart-healthy fats, such as omega-3 fatty acids, which can help reduce inflammation and lower the risk of heart disease. Choosing unsaturated fats aligns with the DASH diet's emphasis on reducing saturated fat intake.

**Low in Added Sugar**: By using fresh berries for sweetness and minimal added sweeteners, this snack keeps added sugar levels low, aligning with the DASH diet's focus on reducing sugar intake.

For individuals adhering to the DASH diet, Greek yogurt with berries is an all-around nutrient-rich and filling snack choice. It offers a harmony of protein, probiotics, vitamins, minerals, antioxidants, and good fats to promote heart health, blood pressure control, and general wellbeing.

# Hummus and Veggie Sticks

The DASH diet's guiding principles are well-aligned with the wholesome and fulfilling snack option of hummus and veggie sticks. This is a thorough explanation:

**Ingredients:**

**Hummus**: Made primarily from chickpeas (garbanzo beans), tahini (sesame seed paste), lemon juice, garlic, and olive oil. It's rich in protein, fiber, healthy fats, vitamins, and minerals.

**Assorted vegetable sticks**: Common choices include carrot sticks, cucumber slices, bell pepper strips, celery sticks, and cherry tomatoes. These provide additional fiber, vitamins (such as vitamin A, vitamin C, and vitamin K), minerals, and antioxidants.

**Preparation:**

Purchase or prepare hummus by blending chickpeas, tahini, lemon juice, garlic, olive oil, and optional seasonings (such as cumin or paprika) until smooth and creamy.

Wash and prepare the vegetables by cutting them into sticks or slices.

Arrange the vegetable sticks on a plate or in a container alongside a serving of hummus.

Serve right away or put in the fridge until you're ready to eat.


**Health Benefits for the DASH Diet:**

**Rich in Fiber**: Hummus and vegetables are both rich in fiber, which supports digestive health, helps control blood sugar levels, and promotes satiety. Adequate fiber intake is an important component of the DASH diet for maintaining overall health and managing blood pressure.

**Heart-Healthy Fats**: Hummus contains heart-healthy fats from olive oil and tahini, which can help lower LDL (bad) cholesterol levels and reduce the risk of heart disease. Choosing unsaturated fats aligns with the DASH diet's emphasis on reducing saturated fat intake.

**Plant-Based Protein**: Chickpeas, the main ingredient in hummus, are a good source of plant-based protein, which supports muscle health, satiety, and overall well-being. Consuming plant-based proteins aligns with the DASH diet's recommendation to include a variety of protein sources in the diet.

**Vitamins and Minerals**: Vegetables provide a variety of vitamins (such as vitamin A, vitamin C, and vitamin K) and minerals (including potassium and magnesium) that contribute to overall health and well-being. Consuming a diverse range of vegetables helps ensure adequate nutrient intake, which is important for managing blood pressure and reducing the risk of chronic diseases.

**Antioxidants**: Both hummus and vegetables contain antioxidants, which help protect cells from damage caused by free radicals and may reduce the risk of chronic diseases such as heart disease and hypertension.

**Low in Added Sugar**: Hummus and vegetables are naturally low in added sugar, making them a suitable option for those following the DASH diet, which emphasizes reducing sugar intake to help manage blood pressure.

# Apple Slices with Almond Butter

Apple slices with almond butter make for a delicious and nutritious snack option that aligns well with the principles of the Dietary Approaches to Stop Hypertension (DASH) diet. Here's a comprehensive explanation:

**Ingredients**:

**Fresh apples**: Provide natural sweetness, fiber, vitamins (such as vitamin C), minerals (including potassium), and antioxidants.
Almond butter: Made from ground almonds, it offers healthy fats, protein, fiber, vitamins (such as vitamin E), minerals (including magnesium and calcium), and antioxidants.

**Preparation**:
Wash the apples thoroughly and slice them into thin wedges or rounds, removing the core and seeds.
Spread a thin layer of almond butter on each apple slice or serve it alongside as a dip.

Optionally, sprinkle the almond butter with cinnamon or a drizzle of honey for added flavor.

Arrange the apple slices on a plate or in a container for serving.

**Health Benefits for the DASH Diet:**

Fiber: Both apples and almond butter are rich in fiber, which supports digestive health, helps control blood sugar levels, and promotes satiety. Adequate fiber intake is an important component of the DASH diet for maintaining overall health and managing blood pressure.

**Healthy Fats**: Almond butter provides heart-healthy monounsaturated fats, which can help lower LDL (bad) cholesterol levels and reduce the risk of heart disease. Choosing unsaturated fats aligns with the DASH diet's emphasis on reducing saturated fat intake.

**Plant-Based Protein**: Almond butter is a good source of plant-based protein, which supports muscle health, satiety, and overall well-being. Consuming plant-based proteins aligns with the DASH diet's recommendation to include a variety of protein sources in the diet.

**Vitamins and Minerals**: Apples and almond butter provide a variety of vitamins (such as vitamin E) and minerals (including potassium, magnesium, and calcium) that contribute to overall health and well-being. Consuming a diverse range of nutrient-rich foods helps ensure adequate nutrient intake, which is important for managing blood pressure and reducing the risk of chronic diseases.

**Antioxidants**: Both apples and almonds contain antioxidants, which help protect cells from damage caused by free radicals and may reduce the risk of chronic diseases such as heart disease and hypertension.

**Low in Added Sugar**: Apples and almond butter are naturally low in added sugar, making them a suitable option for those following the DASH diet, which emphasizes reducing sugar intake to help manage blood pressure.

In conclusion, Apple slices with almond butter are a nutrient-dense and satisfying snack option for those following the DASH diet, providing a balance of fiber, healthy fats, plant-based protein, vitamins, minerals, and antioxidants to support heart health, blood pressure management, and overall well-being.

# CHAPTER SIX

## Incorporating DASH Diet Principles into Your Lifestyle

Incorporating DASH diet principles into your lifestyle can have numerous benefits for your health. Here are some tips on how to do so:

**Increase your intake of fruits and vegetables:** Aim to include a variety of colorful fruits and vegetables in your meals and snacks. These foods are rich in vitamins, minerals, and antioxidants that can help lower blood pressure and reduce the risk of chronic diseases.

**Choose whole grains**: Opt for whole grains such as brown rice, quinoa, whole wheat bread, and oats instead of refined grains. Whole grains are high in fiber, which can help lower cholesterol levels and improve heart health.

**Include lean proteins**: Incorporate lean sources of protein such as poultry, fish, beans, and legumes into your meals. These foods are lower in saturated fat and cholesterol compared to red meat and can help support muscle growth and repair.

**Limit sodium intake:** Reduce your consumption of high-sodium foods such as processed meats, canned soups, and fast food. Instead, season your meals with herbs, spices, and citrus juices to add flavor without the added salt.

**Select healthy fats**: Avoid saturated fats, which are present in butter, cheese, and fatty meats, and choose unsaturated fats, which are found in foods like avocados, nuts, seeds, and olive oil. Good fats have the potential to lessen inflammation and cholesterol levels in the body.

**Practice portion control**: Pay attention to portion sizes and avoid overeating. Use smaller plates, measure out servings, and listen to your body's hunger and fullness cues to prevent overconsumption.

**Keep yourself hydrated**: To maintain general health and stay hydrated, sip lots of water throughout the day. Minimize sugar-filled drinks and substitute them with sparkling water, herbal tea, or water.

You may lower your blood pressure, increase your chances of preventing chronic diseases, and enhance your general health by adopting these DASH diet principles into your daily life. Never forget to speak with a medical professional or qualified nutritionist prior to making any substantial dietary adjustments.

# Dining Out on the DASH Diet

The DASH (Dietary Approaches to Stop Hypertension) diet emphasizes consuming foods rich in nutrients like potassium, calcium, and magnesium while reducing sodium intake. When dining out on the DASH diet, consider these strategies:

**Plan ahead**: Check the restaurant's menu online beforehand to identify DASH-friendly options.

**Choose wisely:** Option for dishes with lean proteins like grilled chicken or fish, plenty of vegetables, whole grains, and fruits.

**Watch portion sizes**: Many restaurants serve oversized portions, so consider sharing a meal or asking for a half-portion.

**Ask for modifications:** Request to have sauces, dressings, and condiments served on the side to control your intake of added sugars and sodium.

**Limit sodium**: Avoid high-sodium foods like processed meats, fried foods, and dishes prepared with lots of salt.

**Stay hydrated**: Drink water or unsweetened beverages instead of sugary sodas or alcoholic drinks.

**Be mindful of cooking methods**: Choose foods that are baked, grilled, steamed, or broiled rather than fried.

**Be cautious with sides:** Option for healthier sides like steamed vegetables, salads with vinaigrette dressing, or a baked potato without excessive toppings.

**Ask questions:** Don't hesitate to inquire about how dishes are prepared and request substitutions or modifications to fit your dietary preferences.

## Smart Snacking Strategies

A dietary regimen called the DASH (Dietary Approaches to Stop Hypertension) diet is intended to help decrease blood pressure and enhance heart health in general. The DASH diet includes smart snacking because it can help control hunger, avoid overindulging during meals, and supply vital nutrients all day long. The following are some wise snacking techniques for the DASH diet:

**Snacks high in nutrients should be chosen**: Go for nutrient-dense snacks including fruits, vegetables, whole grains, nuts, seeds, and lean proteins. Essential vitamins, minerals, and antioxidants included in these foods promote general health.

**Watch portion sizes**: It's important to pay attention to portion sizes when snacking, as overeating can lead to weight gain and other health issues. Aim for smaller portions of snacks that are around 100-200 calories.

**Include a balance of macronutrients**: A balanced snack should include a mix of carbohydrates, protein, and healthy fats to help keep you satisfied and provide sustained energy. For example, pair an apple with a tablespoon of almond butter or a small handful of nuts.

**Limit added sugars and sodium:** Avoid snacks that are high in added sugars and sodium, as these can contribute to high blood pressure and other health problems. Instead, choose whole foods that are naturally low in these additives.

**Plan ahead**: To avoid reaching for unhealthy snacks in a moment of hunger, plan ahead and have nutritious options readily available. Pre-portioned snacks into containers or bags for easy grab-and-go options.

**Listen to your hunger cues**: Pay attention to your body's hunger cues and eat when you are truly hungry, rather than out of boredom or habit. Snack when you need a boost of energy or to tide you over until your next meal.

**Stay hydrated:** Sometimes thirst can be mistaken for hunger, so make sure to stay hydrated throughout the day by drinking plenty of water. Opt for water or unsweetened beverages over sugary drinks.

You may enhance your general health and well-being while adhering to the DASH diet by using these wise snacking practices. To choose nutrient-dense food choices, plan ahead, and pay attention to your body's signals—all of these tips will help you incorporate healthy snacking into your daily routine.

# Tips for Staying on Track

Here are some tips for staying on track with the DASH diet:

**Plan your meals**: One of the keys to success with the DASH diet is planning ahead. Take some time each week to plan out your meals and snacks, making sure to include plenty of fruits, vegetables, whole grains, lean proteins, and low-fat dairy products.

**Stock up on DASH-friendly foods**: Make sure your kitchen is stocked with plenty of DASH-friendly foods, such as fresh fruits and vegetables, whole grains, lean proteins, and low-fat dairy products. Having these healthy options readily available will make it easier to stick to the plan.

**Reduce your sodium intake**: Since the DASH diet is low in sodium, it's critical to watch how much salt you eat. Aim to consume fewer processed foods—which are frequently heavy in sodium—in favor of fresh or minimally processed foods. Instead of using salt to flavor your food, use herbs and spices.

Pay attention to portion sizes because eating too much or even healthy meals can cause weight gain. Try to eat until you are satisfied rather than feeling too full, and pay attention to portion sizes. You can better regulate portion proportions by using smaller bowls and plates.

**Stay hydrated**: Drinking plenty of water is important for overall health and can help you stay on track with the DASH diet. Aim to drink at least eight glasses of water a day, and limit sugary drinks and alcohol.

**Be flexible:** While it's important to follow the guidelines of the DASH diet, it's also important to be flexible and allow yourself some indulgences from time to time. If you have a craving for something that's not on the plan, enjoy it in moderation and then get back on track with your healthy eating.

**Seek support**: Sticking to a new eating plan can be challenging, so don't be afraid to seek support from friends, family, or a healthcare professional. Having someone to hold you accountable and cheer you on can make a big difference in your success with the DASH diet.

You can successfully adhere to the DASH diet and enhance your general health and well-being by using these suggestions and remaining dedicated to your health objectives.

# CHAPTER SEVEN

## DASH Diet FAQs

What is the DASH diet?
The DASH diet is a dietary pattern designed to help lower blood pressure and improve overall health. It emphasizes eating fruits, vegetables, whole grains, lean proteins, and low-fat dairy while limiting sodium, saturated fats, and added sugars.

What are the DASH diet's primary tenets?
The main principles of the DASH diet include increasing intake of fruits, vegetables, whole grains, and low-fat dairy products while reducing consumption of sodium, saturated fats, and added sugars. It also encourages portion control and moderation in alcohol consumption.

Is the DASH diet effective for lowering blood pressure?
Yes, numerous studies have shown that the DASH diet can effectively lower blood pressure, particularly when combined with other lifestyle changes such as regular exercise and weight management.

Can the DASH diet help with weight loss?
While weight loss is not the primary focus of the DASH diet, it can be effective for weight management due to its emphasis on whole, nutrient-rich foods and portion control. However, individual results may vary depending on factors such as calorie intake and physical activity level.

Is the DASH diet suitable for everyone?
The DASH diet is generally considered safe and nutritious for most people, including those with hypertension, diabetes, and other health conditions. However, it's important to consult with a healthcare professional before starting any new diet, especially if you have specific dietary needs or medical concerns.

How can I get started on the DASH diet?
To get started on the DASH diet, begin by gradually incorporating more fruits, vegetables, whole grains, and lean proteins into your meals while reducing sodium, saturated fats, and added sugars. You can also find DASH-friendly recipes and meal plans online or consult with a registered dietitian for personalized guidance.

Are there any potential drawbacks to the DASH diet?
Some people may find it challenging to follow the DASH diet, particularly if they are used to consuming high amounts of sodium, saturated fats, and processed foods. Additionally, individuals with certain dietary restrictions or food allergies may need to modify the diet to meet their needs.

Can I eat out while following the DASH diet?
Yes, you can eat out while following the DASH
diet by making mindful choices, such as
selecting dishes with plenty of vegetables, lean
proteins, and whole grains while avoiding
high-sodium and high-fat options. It's also
helpful to ask about ingredient substitutions
and cooking methods when dining out.

## Overcoming Common Challenges on DASH Diet

Here's a comprehensive guide on how to solve challenges commonly encountered when following the DASH (Dietary Approaches to Stop Hypertension) diet:

**Difficulty reducing sodium intake:**
Reduce the amount of salt that is used at the table and in cooking gradually.
Use herbs, spices, lemon juice, and vinegar to add flavor without extra sodium.
Choose fresh or frozen vegetables and fruits instead of canned ones, as they often contain added salt.
Read food labels carefully and choose products labeled "low sodium" or "no added salt."

**Struggling to incorporate more fruits and vegetables:**
Experiment with different cooking methods such as roasting, grilling, or steaming to enhance flavors.
Try experimenting with new recipes where the main components are fruits and vegetables.
Keep a variety of fruits and vegetables readily available for snacking.
Incorporate fruits and vegetables into dishes like salads, soups, stir-fries, and smoothies.

**Feeling hungry or unsatisfied:**
Prioritize filling, nutrient-dense foods like whole grains, lean proteins, and healthy fats to help you feel fuller for longer.
Eat regular meals and snacks throughout the day to maintain energy levels and prevent overeating.
Pay attention to portion sizes and practice mindful eating, focusing on enjoying each bite and stopping when you feel satisfied.

Stay hydrated by drinking water throughout the day, as thirst can sometimes be mistaken for hunger.

**Difficulty finding DASH-friendly options when eating out:**
Research restaurant menus ahead of time and look for dishes that feature lean proteins, whole grains, and plenty of vegetables.
Ask for modifications or substitutions to make dishes more DASH-friendly, such as requesting dressing on the side or swapping fries for a side salad.
Choose simpler preparations like grilled, steamed, or roasted dishes, and avoid fried or heavily sauced options.
Don't be afraid to ask your server for assistance or recommendations, as many restaurants are willing to accommodate dietary preferences.

**Lack of support or motivation:**
Seek out support from friends, family members, or online communities who are also following the DASH diet. To keep yourself accountable and motivated, set reasonable goals and monitor your progress.
Focus on the positive changes you're making to your health and well-being, rather than dwelling on setbacks.
Consider working with a registered dietitian who can provide personalized guidance, support, and encouragement.

By implementing these strategies, you can overcome common challenges and successfully adhere to the DASH diet for improved health and well-being. Remember that consistency and persistence are key, and don't hesitate to seek support when needed.

# CONCLUSION

In conclusion, embarking on the journey of adopting the DASH (Dietary Approaches to Stop Hypertension) diet can be a transformative step towards achieving better health and overall well-being. The creation of a DASH diet cookbook tailored specifically for beginners serves as an invaluable resource, providing a comprehensive guide and practical tools to navigate the complexities of this dietary approach with confidence and ease.

Through the carefully curated collection of recipes and insightful guidance offered within the pages of a DASH diet cookbook for beginners, individuals are empowered to take control of their health by making informed food choices that promote optimal cardiovascular health and overall wellness. By emphasizing the consumption of nutrient-rich foods such as fruits, vegetables, whole grains, lean proteins, and low-fat dairy products while limiting sodium, saturated fats, and added sugars, the DASH diet offers a balanced and sustainable approach to eating that is both delicious and nourishing.

The cookbook serves as more than just a compilation of recipes; it acts as a comprehensive educational tool, equipping beginners with the knowledge and skills needed to successfully implement the principles of the DASH diet into their daily lives. From practical tips on meal planning and grocery shopping to strategies for dining out and troubleshooting common challenges, the cookbook provides invaluable support every step of the way.

Furthermore, the cookbook recognizes the diverse needs and preferences of individuals embarking on their DASH diet journey, offering a variety of recipes to suit different tastes,

dietary restrictions, and lifestyle factors.
Whether craving a hearty and comforting meal,
a light and refreshing snack, or a decadent yet
health-conscious dessert, there is something
for everyone within the pages of the cookbook.

Ultimately, the DASH diet cookbook for
beginners serves as a beacon of hope and
empowerment, guiding individuals towards a
healthier and happier future. By embracing the
principles of the DASH diet and incorporating
flavorful and nourishing recipes into their daily
routine, beginners can embark on a
transformative journey towards better health,
reduced risk of chronic disease, and improved
quality of life. With dedication, perseverance,
and the support of a trusted resource like the
DASH diet cookbook for beginners, individuals
can achieve their health goals and experience
the countless benefits of this evidence-based
dietary approach for years to come.

Thank you for taking the time to explore the DASH Diet Cookbook. We hope you found the recipes and information within its pages inspiring and helpful on your journey to better health. By embracing the principles of the DASH diet and incorporating these delicious and nutritious recipes into your daily routine, you're taking proactive steps towards a healthier lifestyle. Keep in mind that even minor adjustments might have a big impact on your general wellbeing. We appreciate your support and interest, and as you start this delicious and rewarding journey with us, we look forward to hearing about your accomplishments. To your well-being, cheers!

www.ingramcontent.com/pod-product-compliance
Lightning Source LLC
Chambersburg PA
CBHW070950250726
48663CB00002B/159